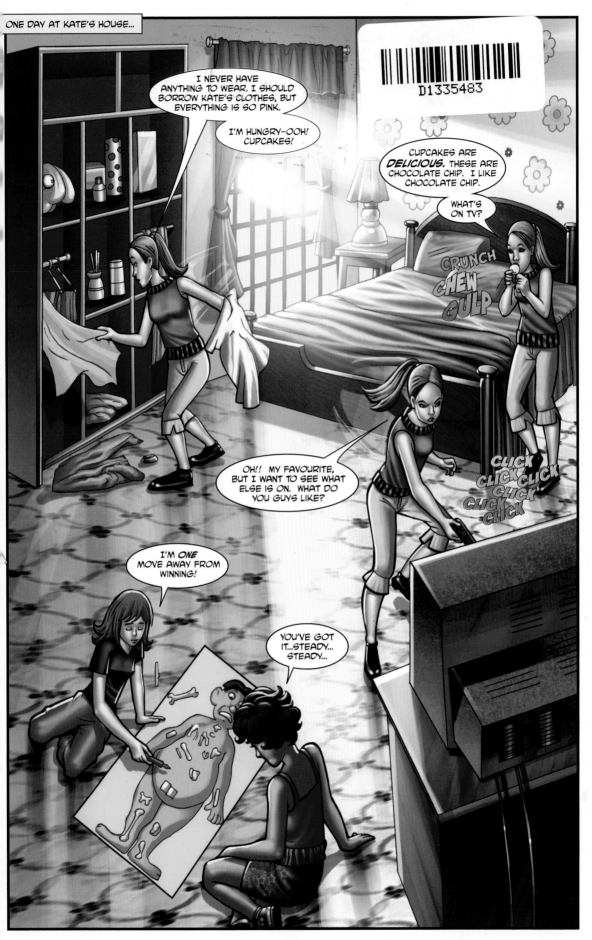

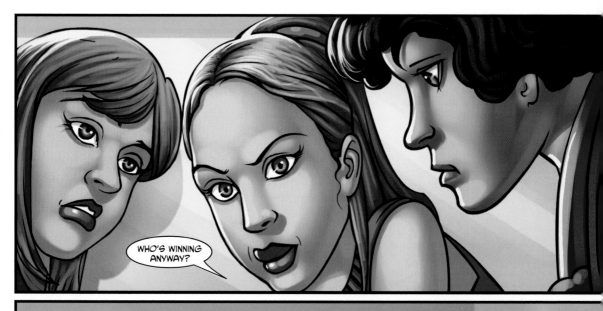

WHO'S WINNING ANYWAY?

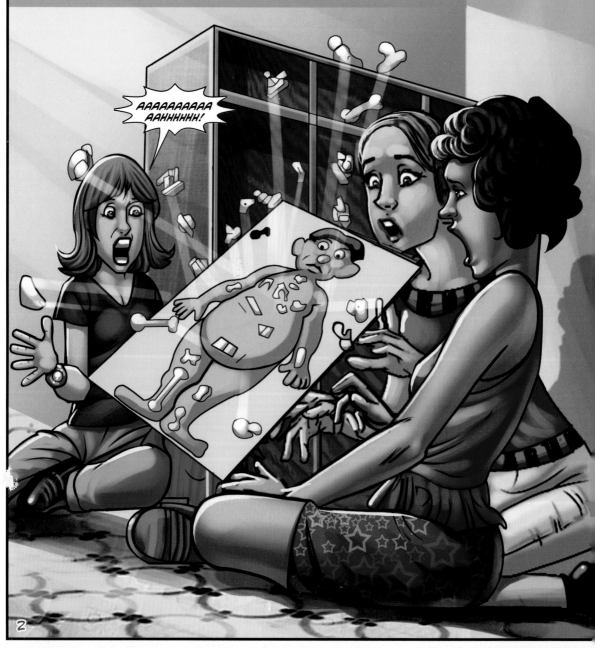

AAAAAAAAAA AAHHHHHH!

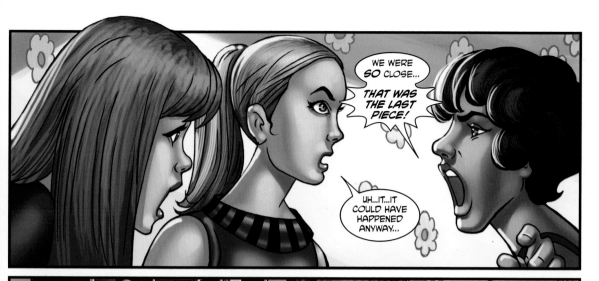

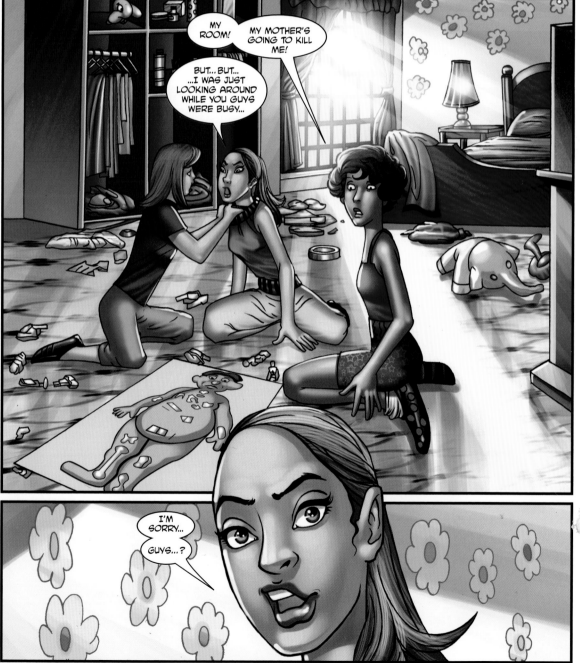

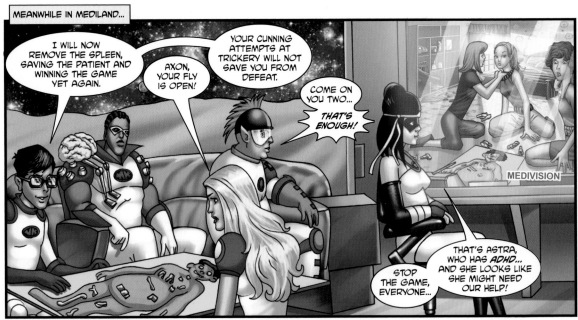

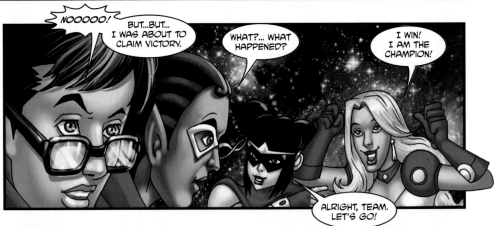

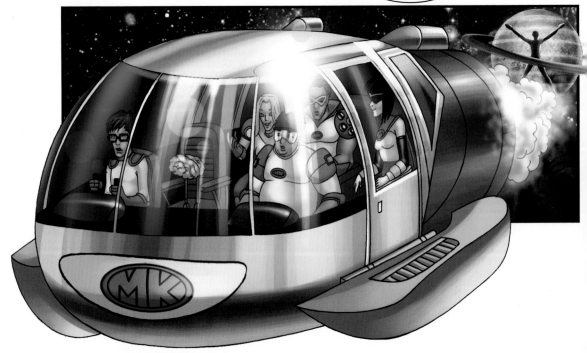

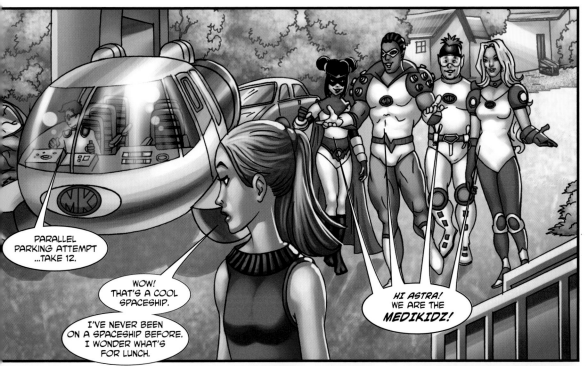

PARALLEL PARKING ATTEMPT ...TAKE 12.

WOW! THAT'S A COOL SPACESHIP.

I'VE NEVER BEEN ON A SPACESHIP BEFORE. I WONDER WHAT'S FOR LUNCH.

HI ASTRA! WE ARE THE MEDIKIDZ!

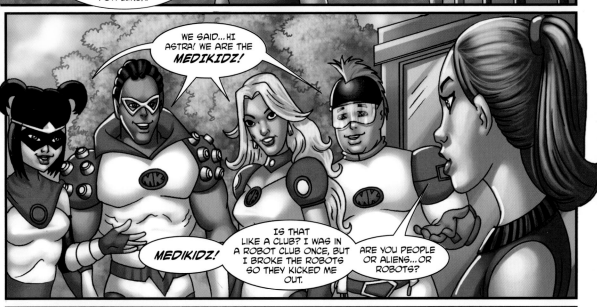

WE SAID... HI ASTRA! WE ARE THE MEDIKIDZ!

MEDIKIDZ!

IS THAT LIKE A CLUB? I WAS IN A ROBOT CLUB ONCE, BUT I BROKE THE ROBOTS SO THEY KICKED ME OUT.

ARE YOU PEOPLE OR ALIENS...OR ROBOTS?

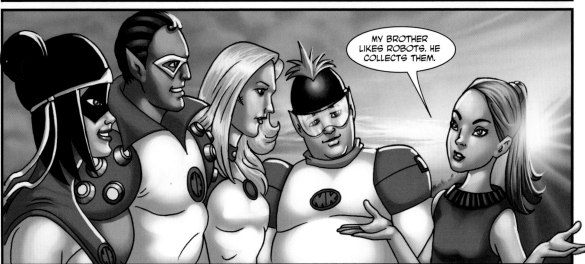

MY BROTHER LIKES ROBOTS. HE COLLECTS THEM.

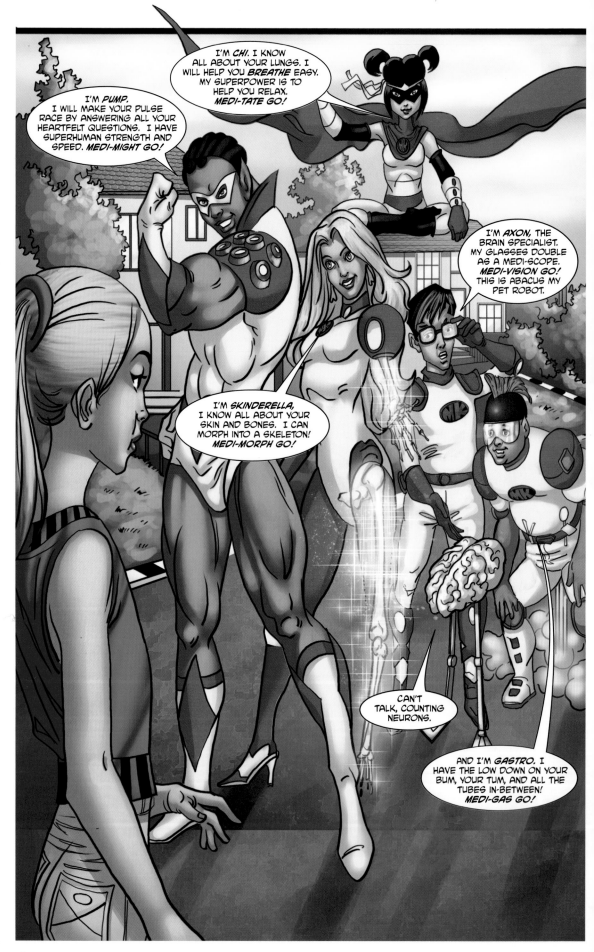

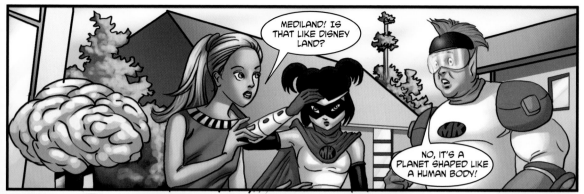

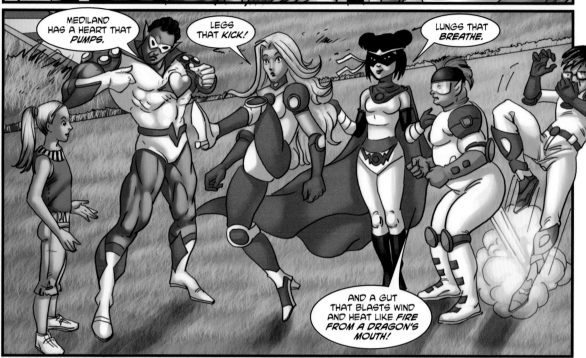

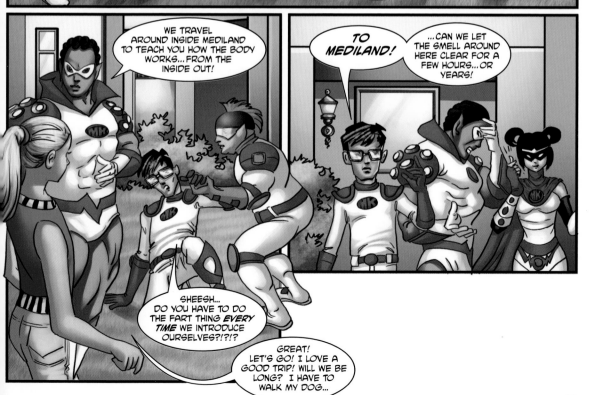

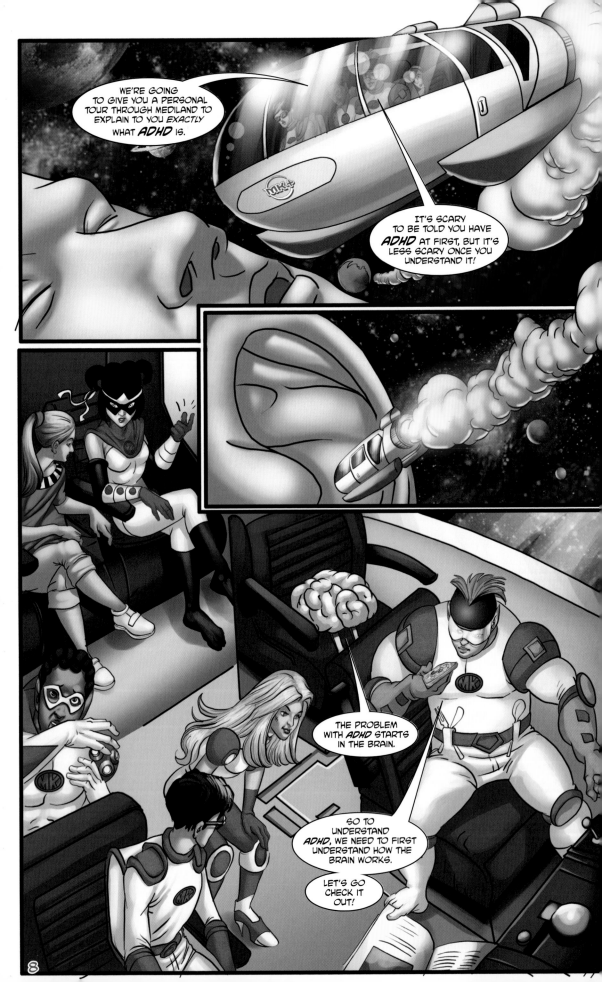

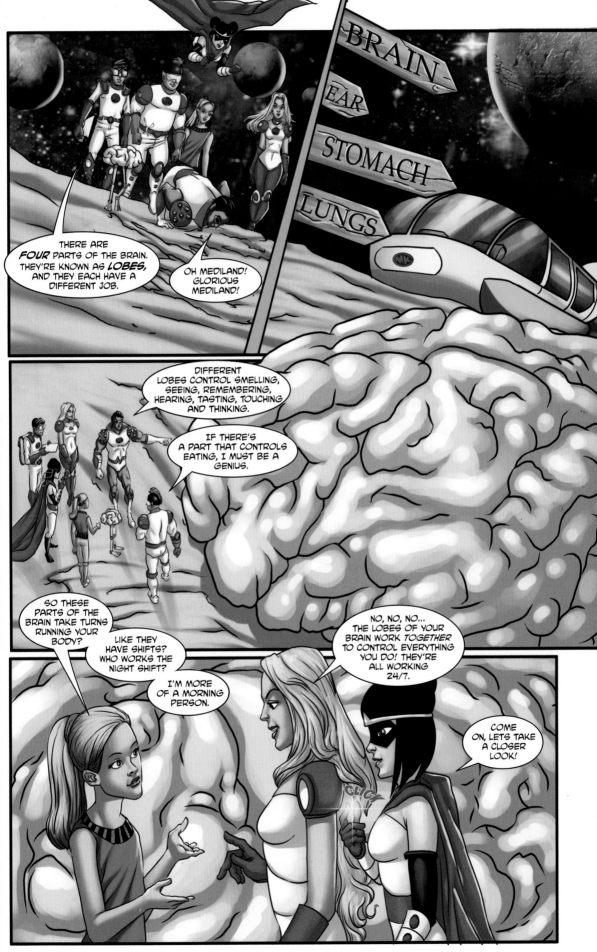

THERE ARE *FOUR* PARTS OF THE BRAIN. THEY'RE KNOWN AS *LOBES*, AND THEY EACH HAVE A DIFFERENT JOB.

OH MEDILAND! GLORIOUS MEDILAND!

BRAIN

EAR

STOMACH

LUNGS

DIFFERENT LOBES CONTROL SMELLING, SEEING, REMEMBERING, HEARING, TASTING, TOUCHING AND THINKING.

IF THERE'S A PART THAT CONTROLS EATING, I MUST BE A GENIUS.

SO THESE PARTS OF THE BRAIN TAKE TURNS RUNNING YOUR BODY?

LIKE THEY HAVE SHIFTS? WHO WORKS THE NIGHT SHIFT?

I'M MORE OF A MORNING PERSON.

NO, NO, NO... THE LOBES OF YOUR BRAIN WORK *TOGETHER* TO CONTROL EVERYTHING YOU DO! THEY'RE ALL WORKING 24/7.

COME ON, LETS TAKE A CLOSER LOOK!

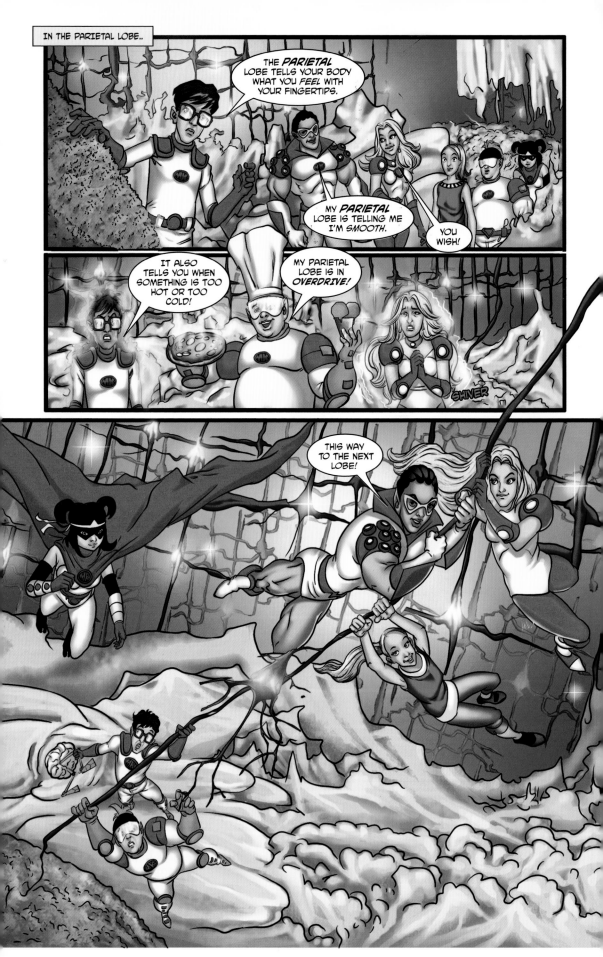

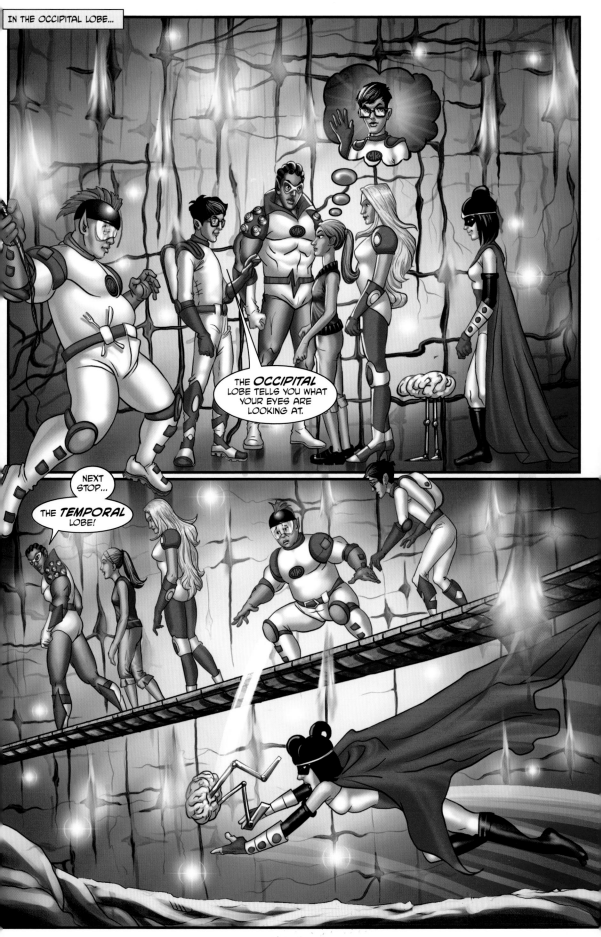

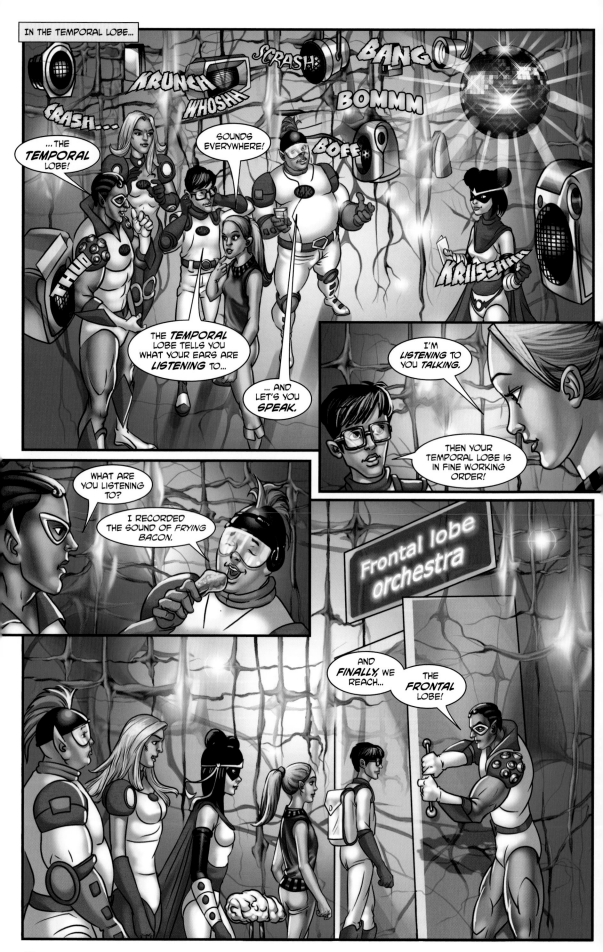

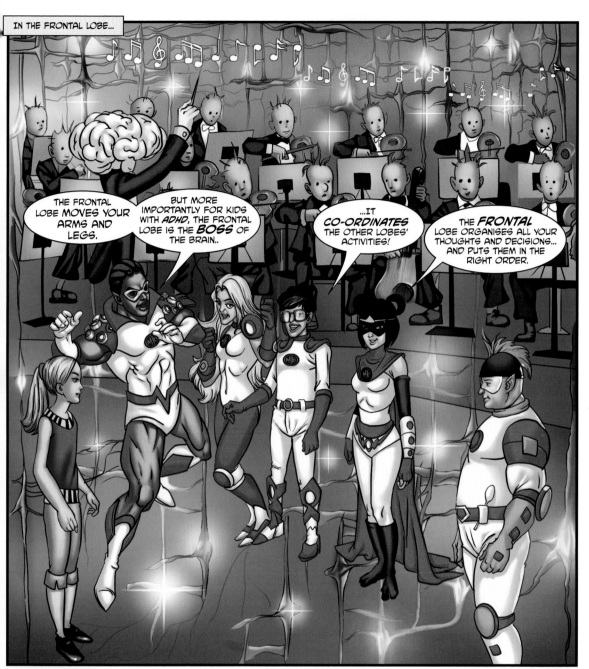

THE FRONTAL LOBE MOVES YOUR ARMS AND LEGS.

BUT MORE IMPORTANTLY FOR KIDS WITH *ADHD*, THE FRONTAL LOBE IS THE *BOSS* OF THE BRAIN..

...IT *CO-ORDINATES* THE OTHER LOBES' ACTIVITIES!

THE *FRONTAL* LOBE ORGANISES ALL YOUR THOUGHTS AND DECISIONS... AND PUTS THEM IN THE RIGHT ORDER.

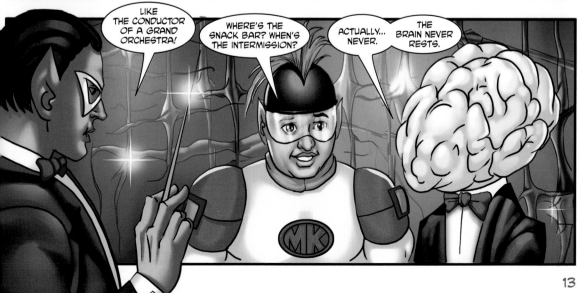

LIKE THE CONDUCTOR OF A GRAND ORCHESTRA!

WHERE'S THE SNACK BAR? WHEN'S THE INTERMISSION?

ACTUALLY... NEVER.

THE BRAIN NEVER RESTS.

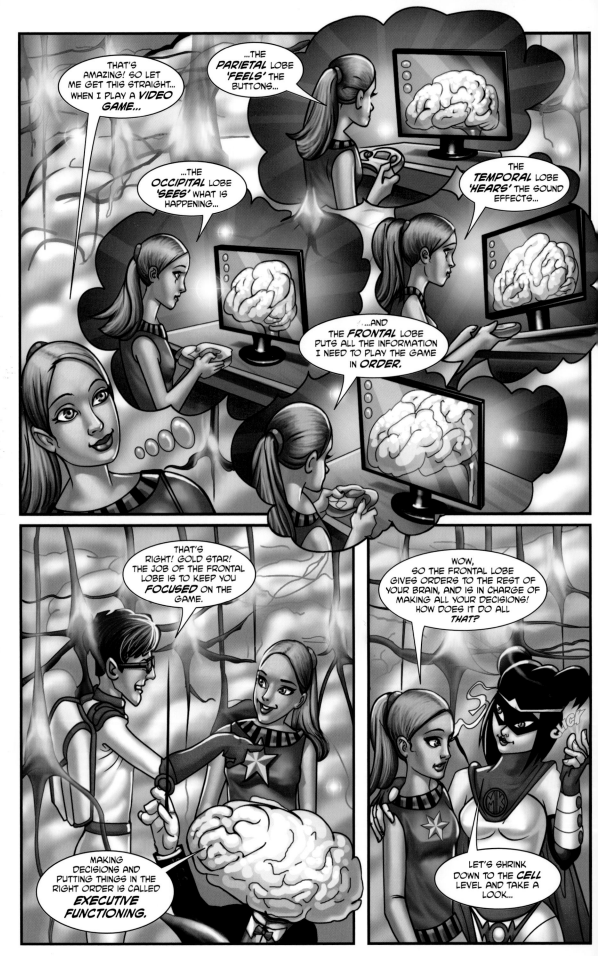

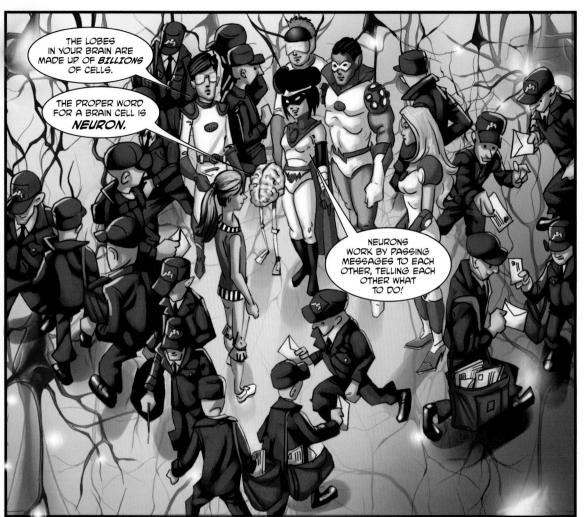

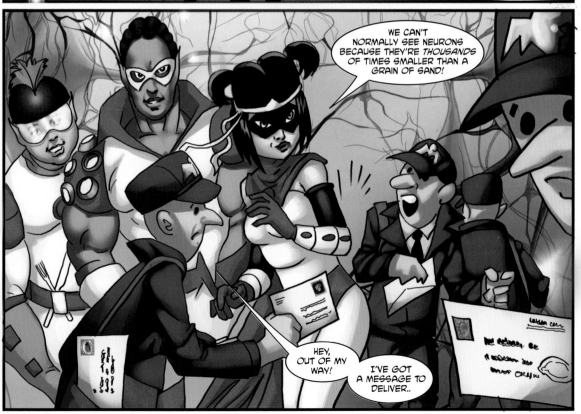

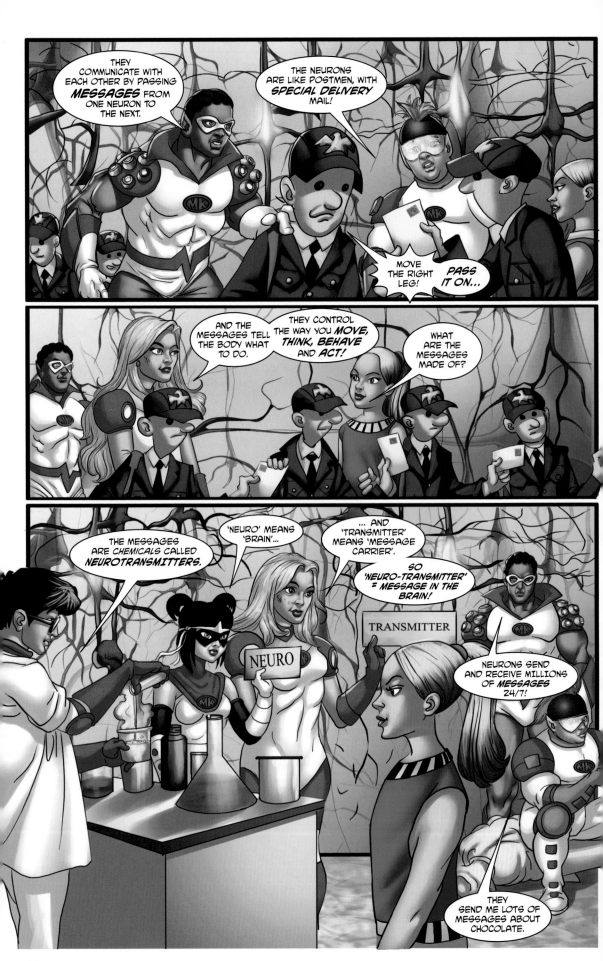

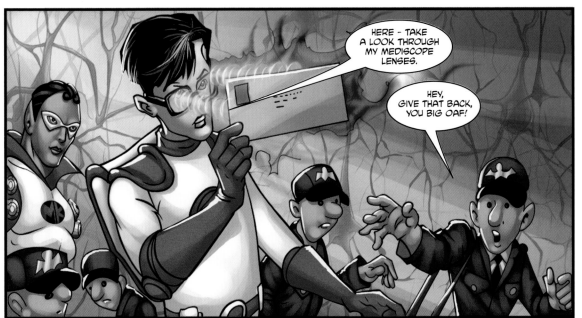

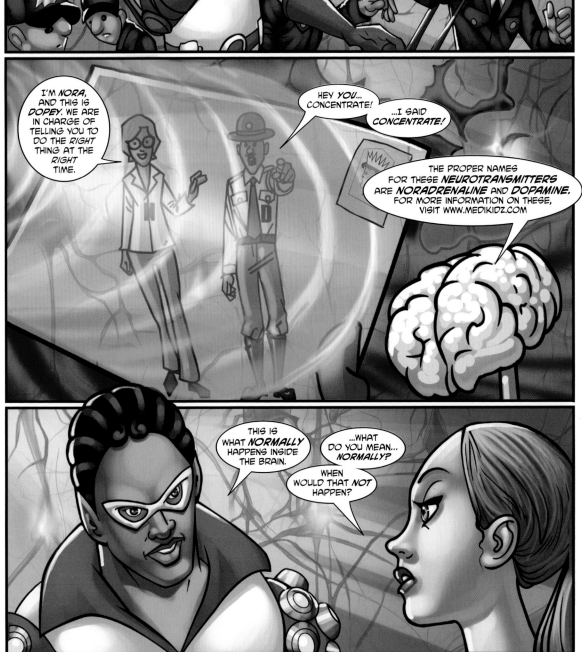

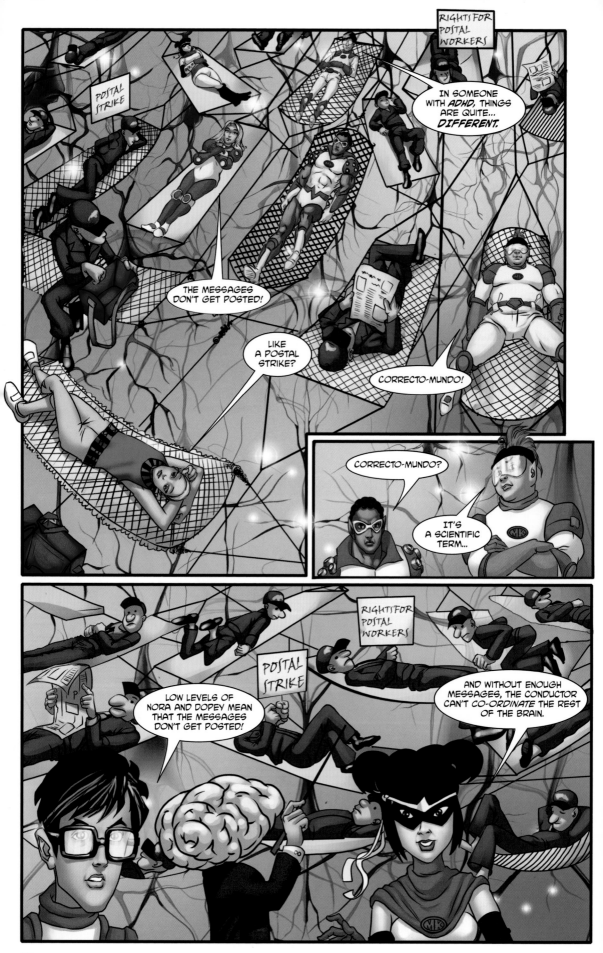

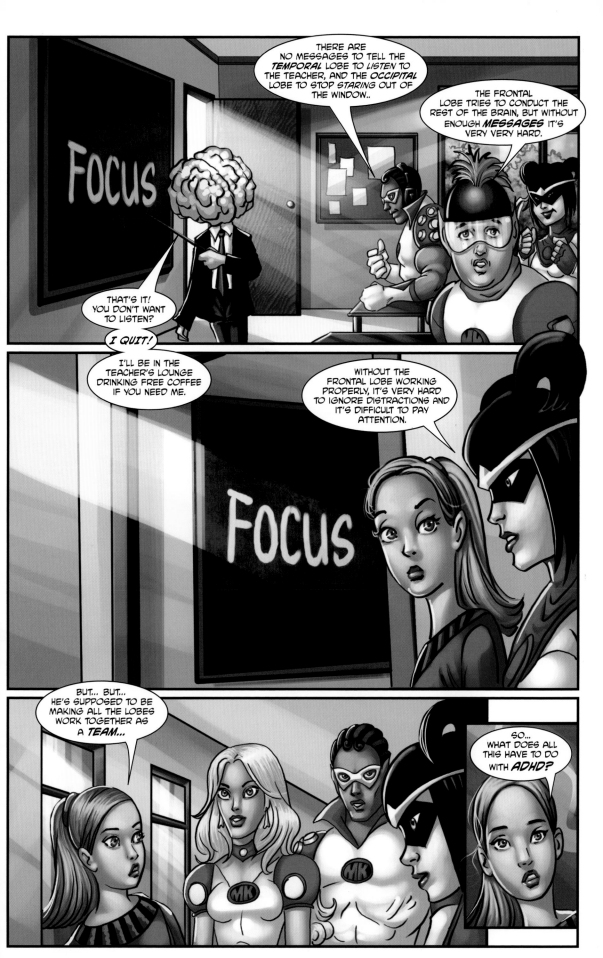

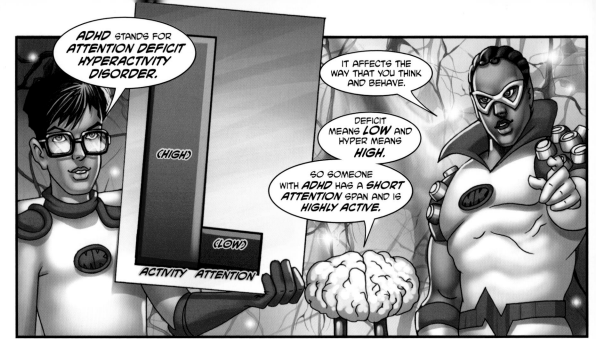

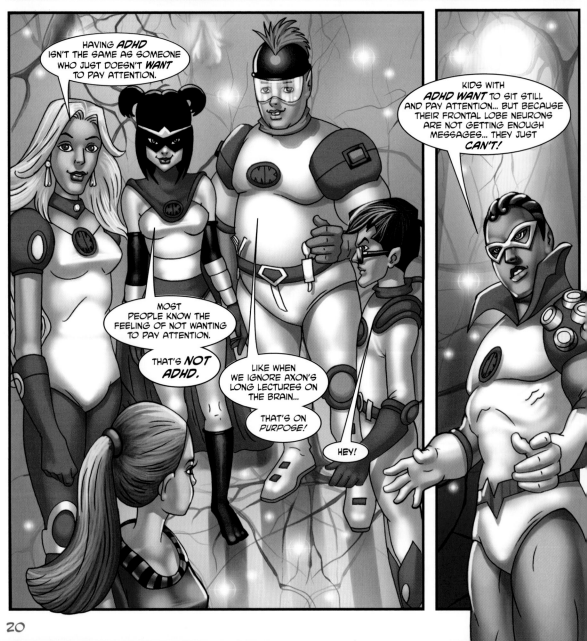

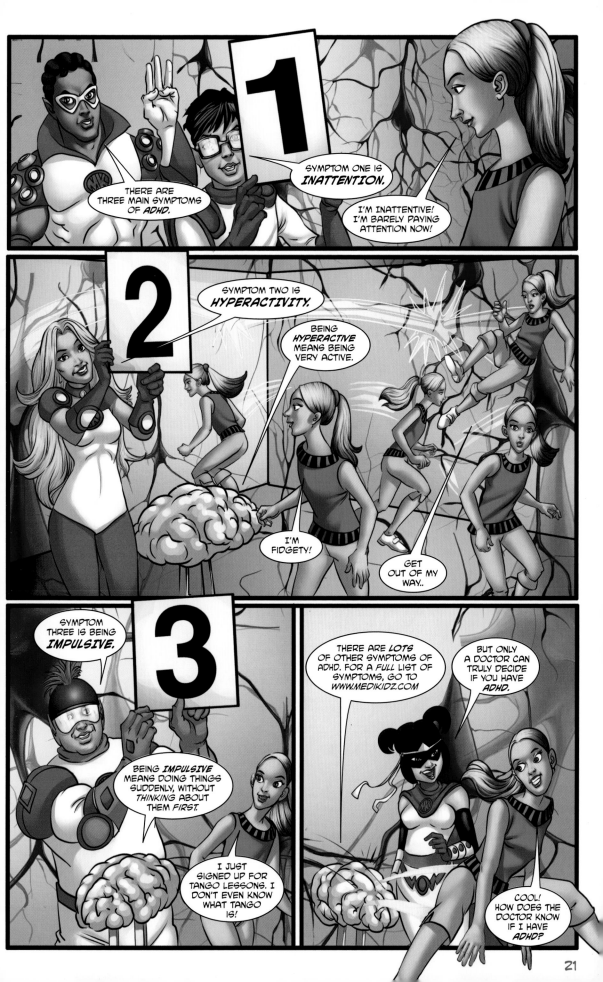

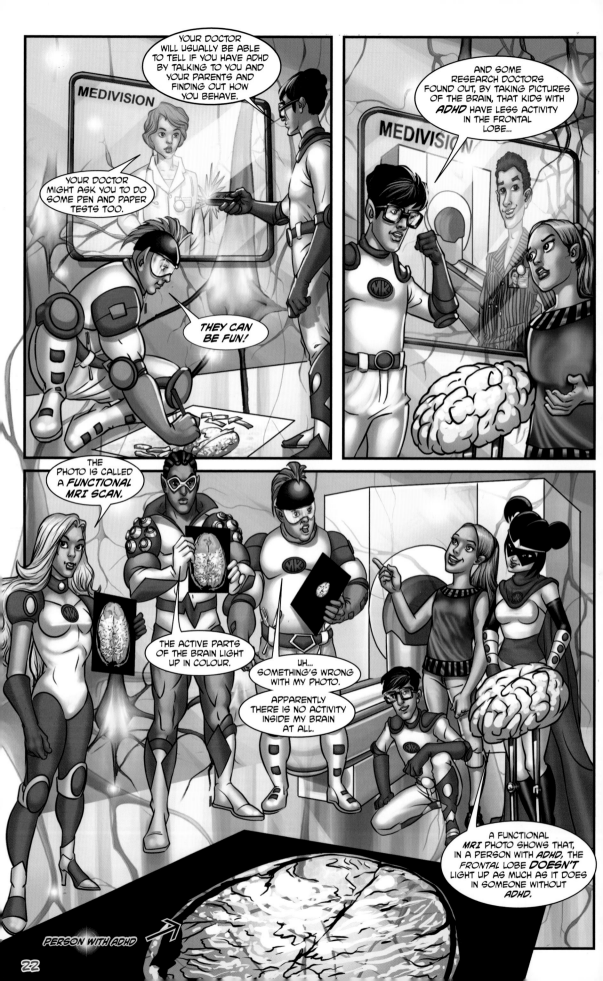

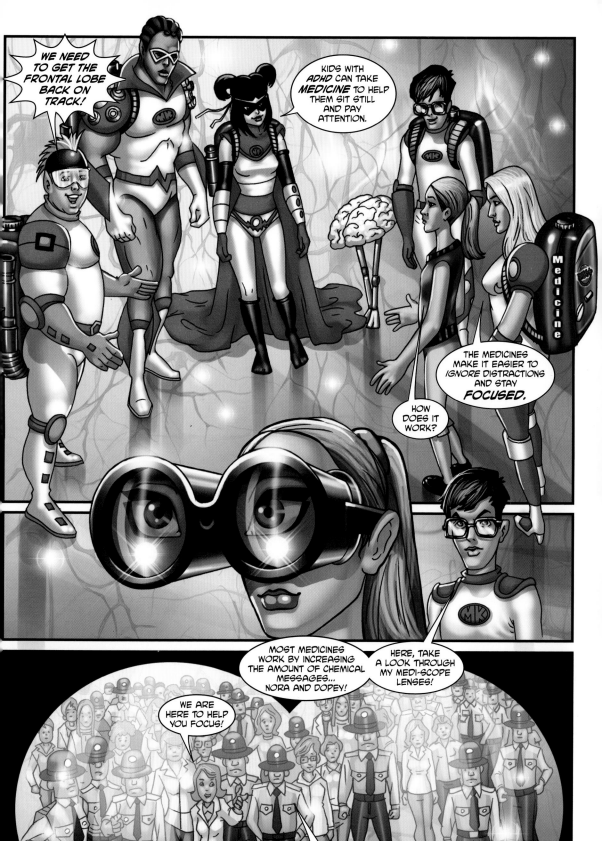

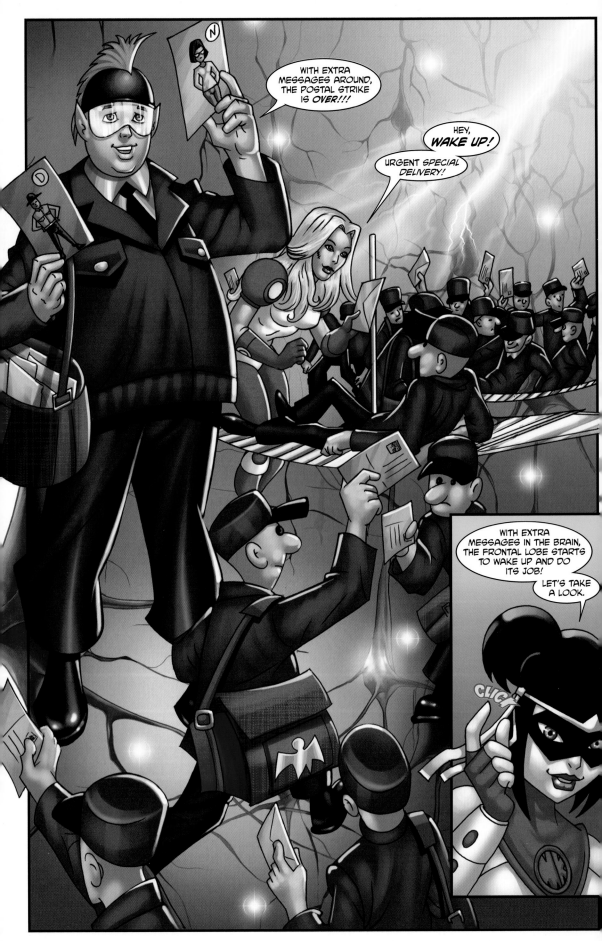

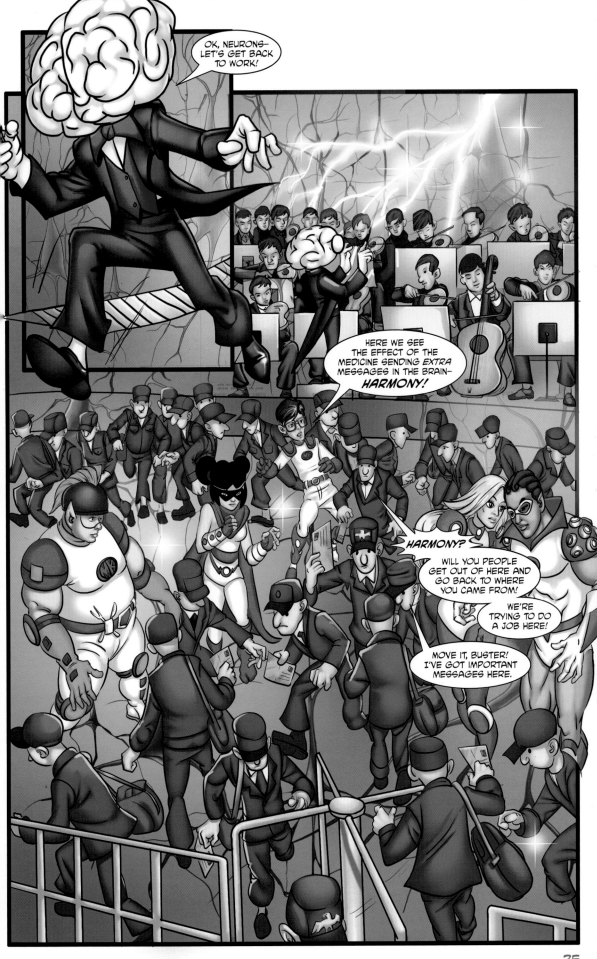

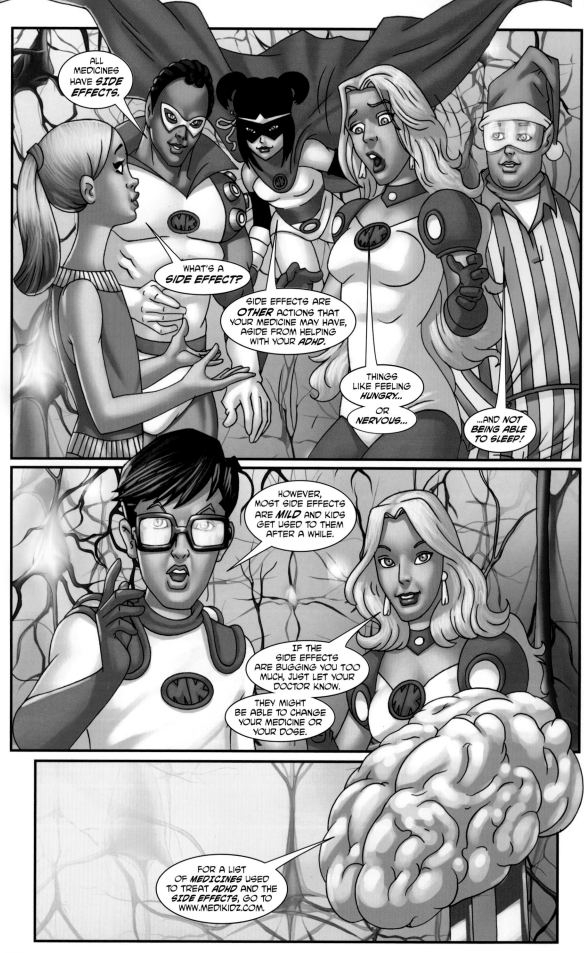

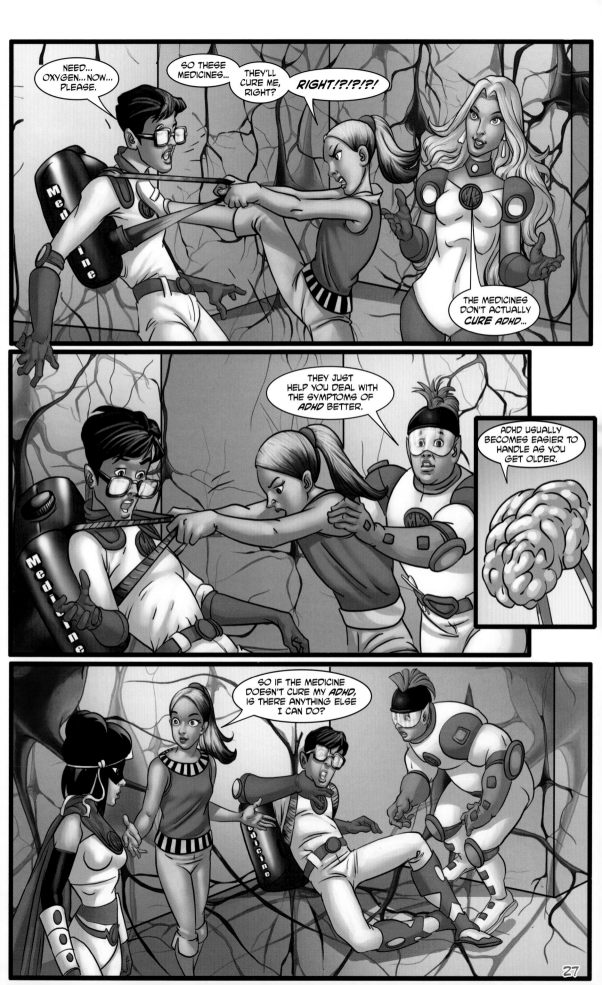

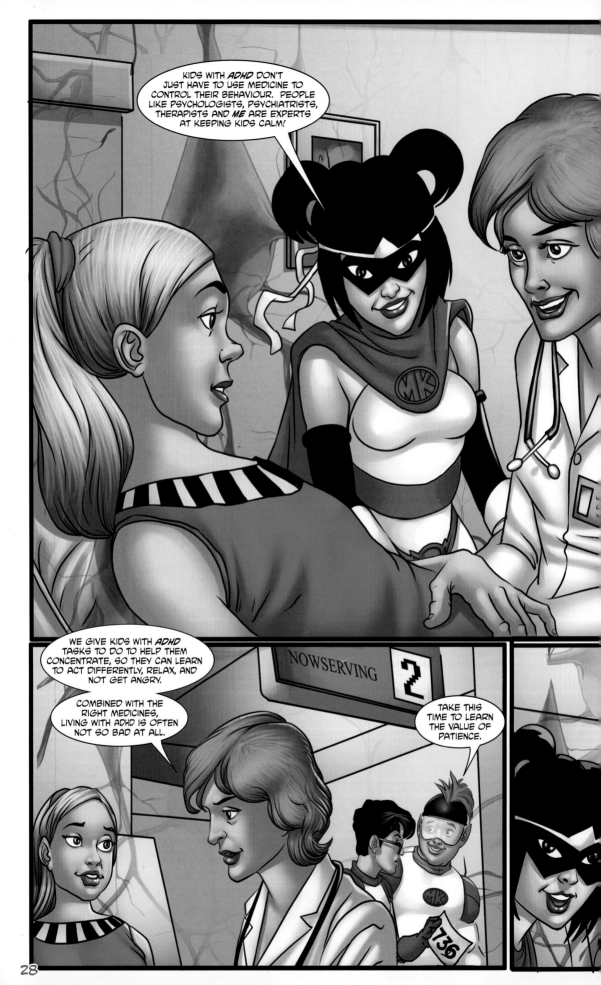

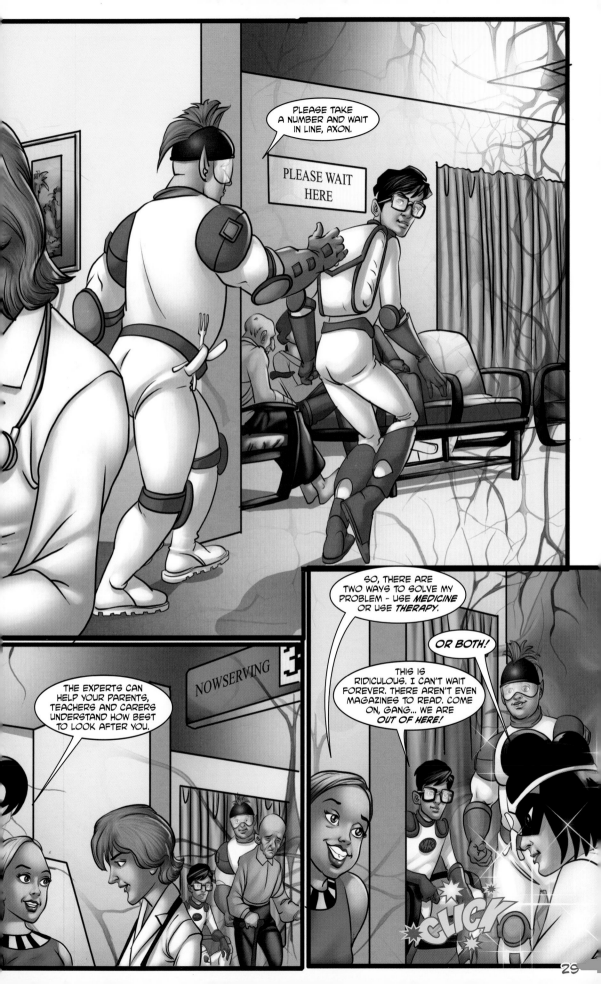

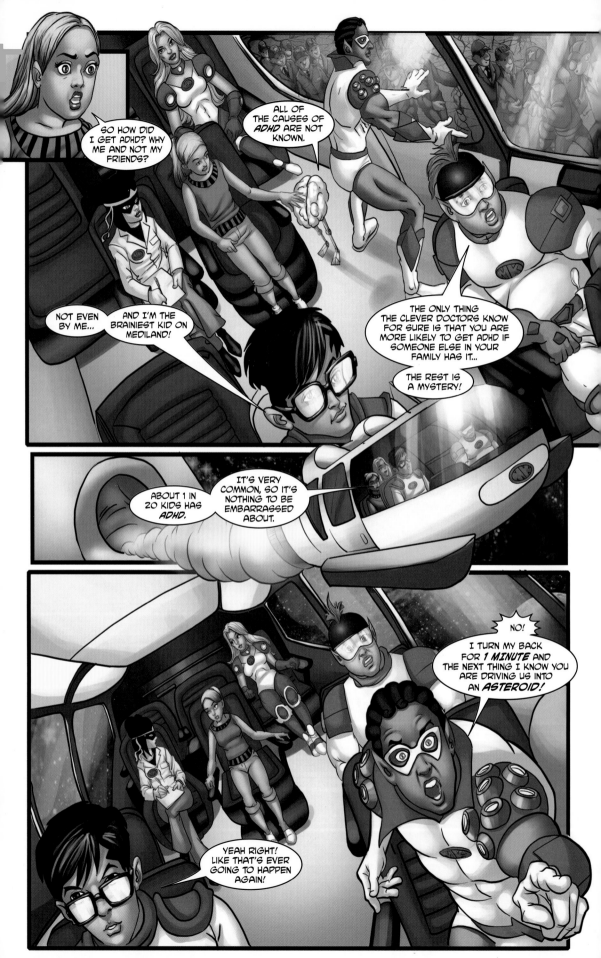

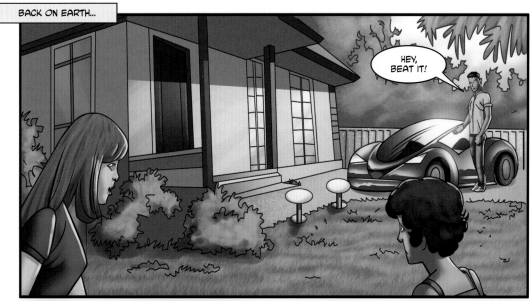

HEY, BEAT IT!

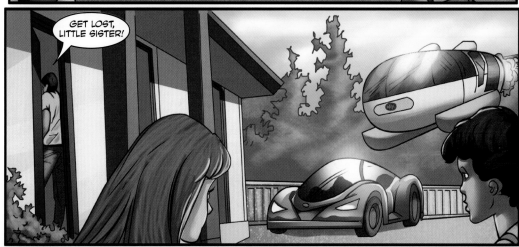

GET LOST, LITTLE SISTER!

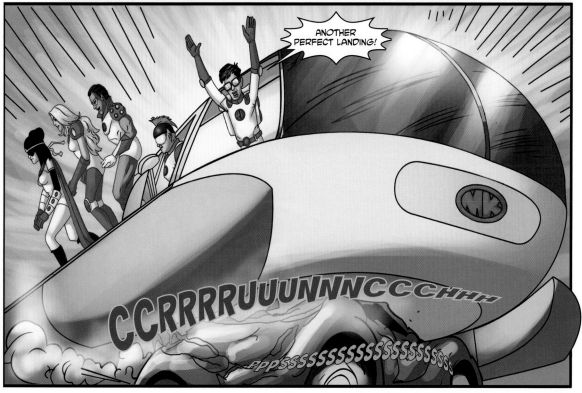

ANOTHER PERFECT LANDING!

CCRRRRUUUNNNCCCHHH

PPPSSSSSSSSSSSSSSSSSSSSS

31

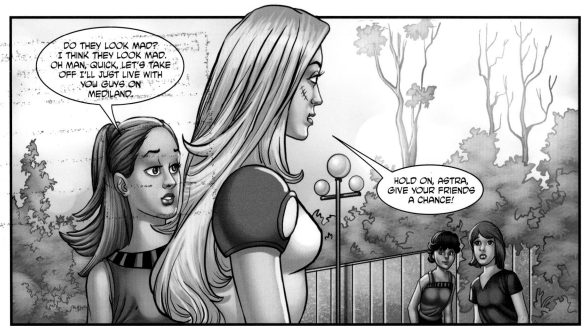

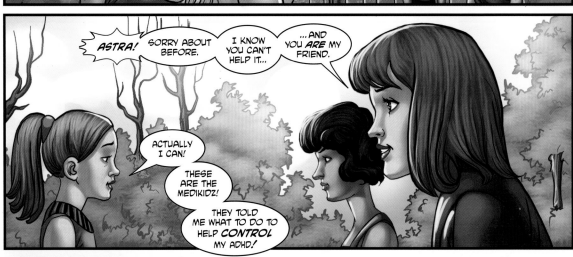

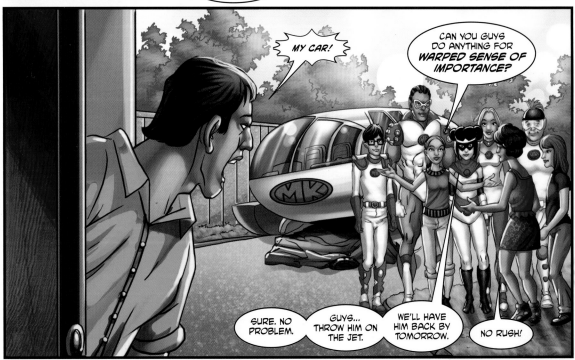